PAIN:
Therapies & Treatments

Ariele M. Huff

DEDICATION

To all those who have shared remedies that have helped me.

CONTENTS

Introduction

Ariele M. Huff

INTRODUCTION

Dear Reader, fellow human, friend: I have experienced many kinds of intense physical pain from the thigh to ankle bone-deep cut at 22 months old to migraines, unmedicated childbirth, kidney stones, shingles, injuries from five accidents—four car and one motorcycle, death of tooth nerves, root canals, extractions, chronic acid reflux, a fibroid entrapped ovary, and arthritis among others. As a result, I have a handful of powerful and amazing strategies and techniques to share. I believe you will find something in this book that will help you. (I am not a doctor or health care provider. Aside from being a sufferer like you, I have worked at a Sports Medicine and a Naturopathic clinic. Dr. Bastyr for whom the Naturopathic College and Clinic in Seattle were named was my doctor for 23 years and taught me many strategies for pain relief. Of course, you should check out any of the physical therapies with your doctor. I love the fact that many of these methods are mental ways to alter, modify, or eliminate pain and can be utilized safely by anyone.)

Pain is a Friend

Like an alarm clock that wakes us up or a smoke alarm that gets us out of the house, pain is a gift and a friend. Physical and emotional pains are signals to do something that, if ignored, become more intense. As a writing instructor, I've come to believe one of the most universal human needs is to be heard. Similarly, your pain wants recognition and attention. It always arrives with an important message. To find patterns in your pain, document when it happens—what foods, activities, medications, or emotions might be associated with its occurrences. Once patterns are discovered, you are able to experiment with changes that may short circuit the pain reaction even before it starts. Prevention is the happiest cure of all!

The Wonders of Witnessing

When dealing with physical and emotional pain and fear, this strategy neighbors on miraculous. The instructions are simple; the effect profound. I learned witnessing by stumbling onto it while coping with an acute fear. It is taught in many mindfulness practices: yoga, Tai Chi, Qigong, etc.

+ First, go to a spot where you won't be interrupted. Do this process alone the first few times, at least, as focus is required.

+ Put your awareness, your attention on the pain.

+ Then, allow yourself to feel the pain without doing anything to stop it, to resent it, to fear it, or to change it. Just notice it. Allow it to be. Allow yourself to be with it. The effect of simply placing attention on a pain or fear can, sometimes, eliminate it instantly. I have experienced that with migraines, tight muscles, and dental pain. An entrenched discomfort often undergoes a change—location, intensity, type of sensation—pressure, itching, heat/cold, or other sensations may replace sharp pain. Sometimes, it takes a few minutes for the emotional self to process the physical alteration, to believe it has happened. Even pain that is part of an ongoing situation—a wound, a disease process, a dysfunctional part—can become more like "distant thunder" than like an ever present screaming smoke alarm. The resulting relief allows better sleep, less stress—promoting better healing or coping with conditions. When you get good at this practice, you'll be able to do it anywhere.

Relaxation

Several relaxation techniques are part of my first aid kit for pain. Often, some deep breaths or the yogic exercise of inhaling for 4 counts, holding for 7, exhaling strongly for 8 are enough. Sometimes, progressive relaxation (telling my body to relax a part at a time) does the trick. Doing the trick means I can feel my shoulders dropping and my face/solar plexus/diaphragm relaxing, or I fall asleep. Other times, I need some external help. My top favorite is *Letting Go of Stress*, a CD by Emmett Miller, MD and Steven Halpern that has "four effective techniques for relaxation and stress reduction." My favorite is the one with the elevator, but they are all good. I've brought this in to listen to through earphones during root canals. The first time, I was so relaxed that my dentist thought I'd fallen asleep or passed out. Neither, though I wasn't far from sleep! When I know I'll be anxious— before a surgery or procedure, for example, I often prepare by associating the experience with a really pleasant one, establish a "trigger" place to tap on my hand or leg, and...voila...I'm smiling and not tense as I walk in. This has absolutely led me to have less pain after surgeries and procedures.

Releasing

Releasing is a good follow up to witnessing or a good practice to use on a daily basis as issues arise. We all do some natural releasing of emotions and physical feelings, but techniques like Sedona Releasing have taught me that any situation can profit from this method—even those conditions that seem most unrelenting. As with witnessing, this is best done alone initially. Find your discomfort again. Visualize the discomfort. Is it a cloud or a knife or a heavy hand or something else? See an image of it. Allow the image to exit your body as something quick moving, like steam from a kettle or a flow of energy or as wind whistling out of a tunnel. A good exit point for generalized body discomfort can be the stomach or chest, but finding specific spots on the body and visuals to go with each is also effective. Continue watching this as long as it takes to have an alteration...often feeling lighter. Once release starts, do check in with the area mentally and purposely soften and relax it. With some arising pain, releasing can be done quite quickly. Images I like are oil gushing from an oil well or a dog shaking the water off its coat. Quick movement. Releasing during movement—running or swimming—has been especially powerful. Releasing out in a natural spot has also added to the impact of the process for me.

Positive Pictures

A positive picture shows a health goal with words that describe it as having been achieved. I often find a way to personify body parts that are involved—my heart as a nervous little baby pig I held and calmed in my arms, my esophagus an angry snake rising from my stomach to my throat and being reassured it was listened and cared for. I use colors to add power. The important thing is that the picture puts you into your desired situation, and demonstrates what it will look and sound like once you've gotten what you want. Use positive words.

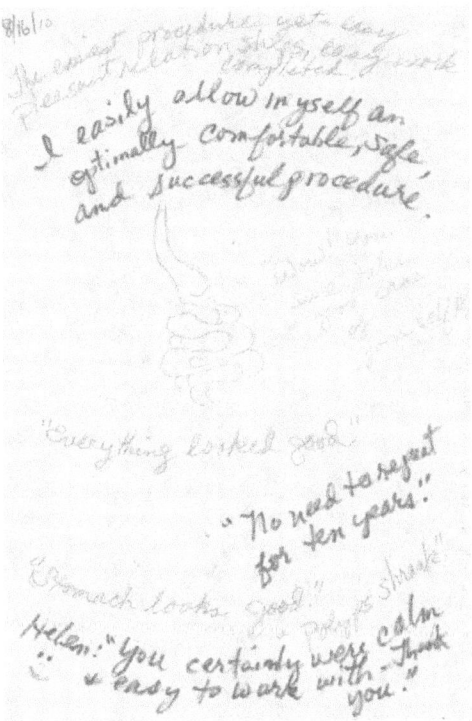

This picture was created to prepare for an upper endoscopy/colonoscopy. A drawing of my digestive system is surrounded by optimistic outcomes about the ease of the procedure, my comfort, and the quotes of those around me praising my behavior and health. Note the specifics like "polyps shrank" and "no need to repeat for ten years." While both of those were unlikely and did not happen, I include any optimal results I'd like to have. Why not? Even some of those have come true—against all odds. I have done these for most of my life.

Moving the Golden Light

For healing: Feel the life energy in your hands—pulsating, buzzing, tingling. See that as a light and move it to whatever spot is injured or ill. Holding a hand over the spot can be useful or focusing a light bulb on it. Experiencing the tingling and bright light in movement—sweeping back and forth or circulating around a spot, or from head to toe—can be really potent. During healing, I've spent hours doing this successfully. It often requires several days. However, the body naturally does this for injuries. I especially noticed this when I had a cut or burn to my hands. The life energy was rushed to that area. Well, I thought, if the healing can be felt in the fingers and hands, then it can happen anywhere. I've now used it in many areas and for many issues. The practice, called moving the Golden Flower, was taught to me by my parents when I was a child. They raised us (sister and me) doing yoga and meditation. My most stunning success with this took several hours with a light bulb focussed on the area of a painful ovarian cyst which resolved as a result.

Energy Healing

While I've heard that this is something non-professionals can do for each other, I had an exceptional healer treat me after a bad whiplash accident that was magnifying the complications of four previous accidents. (I have to say: None were my fault. I was a passenger in two of them and struck from the side by vehicles illegally emerging from side streets or a parking lot outside my line of vision.) At any rate, the Energy Healing was done by a woman who mostly did not touch me, but I could feel the warmth and buzzing energy from her hands. I recognize that some will think of this as "woo woo," but, what can I say? I felt it with my eyes shut and, most significantly, it absolutely helped me with pain that was resistant to all other approaches. I wish for you that you can find someone as good. Beware of fakes, of course. My practitioner was operating out of a doctors' clinic, was a certified masseuse and physical therapist, and had diplomas all over her walls. Another therapy that has helped me, though less amazing, is Trigger Point massage. I've also had some good effects from acupuncture, though—after years of it—I can no longer tolerate the needles. (Note that Japanese acupuncture uses electrical stimulation at the points and is not painful at all.) Chiropractic has also helped me at some times, but as I age, I am more careful about that or regular massage techniques as I'm likely to find myself in more pain after those treatments than before them. This is one of the reasons why mental forms of pain modification and elimination are such awesome discoveries for me. And, yes, I can use those methods to help me get through things I feel will eventually help even if they cause increased pain or symptoms—surgeries, dental procedures, chiropractic, physical therapies, etc.

Love and Approval

Three more dynamic exercises come from the Releasing method. These strategies often work when others haven't completely, especially if any anger, denial, or frustrations are present.

+ Try this: Go to the area of discomfort or dysfunction. Say, "yes" to that place in you, accepting it without judgment. Repeat until you feel a change.

+ Another exercise: Send approval to any bodily or emotional place that is uncomfortable or negative. Approval can be simply visualized as an audience clapping, a smiling facing, being presented with an award, being patted on the back, or being in a hugging circle.

+ And finally: Send love to any bodily part that is having trouble. My favorite way to start this process is to visualize someone I love a lot. The feeling that floods me is strong, tender, and affectionate. Happily, we can borrow on our better love of another person to help ourselves. (FYI—it works to visualize a beloved pet too.)

Meditation and Yoga

Not to be left out, meditation is broadly known to help with pain management and relief. Unlike the methods already mentioned, meditation brings relaxation, clarity, and healing to the whole self—without any particular focus on specific components or issues. It is also an excellent background for all the other practices mentioned. Meditation makes minds, intuitions, and bodies operate more efficiently. Combining this with whatever level or kind of yoga you can tolerate will enhance the benefits of each. (Most people can do some yoga—breathing exercises and gentle stretches, for example. Kundalini yoga involves a lot of work with the inner energy system—including moving the Golden Flower— that can even be done by a person with paralysis.)

The Role of Diet

What we nourish our bodies with can't be underestimated as affecting the physical and emotional aspects of ourselves. Many fine books exist on diets for every kind of illness or state of recovery from injury. However, some of these do not go far enough for maximum benefit. In other words, they play to our hope that we can eat and drink what we want and still get healthier. Here are a few things I've learned in the process of modifying pain and causes of it.

+ Sugar in any form (yes, including alcohol) is the worst enemy of any pain relief plan.

+ Processed foods offer little of value (nutrients) and a lot of things that are hard on the body (excess salt, saturated fat, sugar, chemicals, fillers). Pain is a signal that the body needs all its resources to create a better condition. That means the closest to natural foods that we can get.

+ Lean protein—plant or animal should be present at each meal.

+ Small meals are best, spread through the day.

+ My famous naturopath, Dr. Bastyr, said that no one should eat after 4 pm.

+ I find that a diet rich in vegetables makes me feel better. When I'm weak or having digestive discomfort, cooked vegetables are gentler. Brief steaming or sautéing leaves most of the nutrients intact.

+ Stay hydrated. Some fluids are dehydrating: coffee, tea, caffeinated soda. Some contain too much sugar: juices and commercially produced smoothies. Some foods are hydrating: watermelon, cucumbers, and light soups and broths, for instance.

+ Fresh herbs like rosemary, thyme, sage, lavender, and oregano are easy to grow and have traditionally been used to cure diseases. Ditto for some spices like cinnamon and turmeric.

+ Eat less. Studies show that people live longer and are healthier when they eat less than most people do.

+ Experiment to discover which healthy foods you like and ways to prepare them that are enjoyable to you.

Water Therapies

My parents and Dr. Bastyr were all impressed with how effective the use of water could be. In my difficult peri-pause (time going into menopause when I had a fibroid painfully wrapped around an ovary), I used an Epsom salts bath daily. Dr. Bastyr said to make the water "as hot as you can stand," then "stay in it until it cools down to the point where you need to get out of it." This was highly successful in relaxing the area and freeing me temporarily of the pain. I did get the surgery later. Do be aware that this process brings up the blood pressure for a short while after the bath. (I've read that some experts say transitory raises like that can be good for moderating bp, but not for someone who tends to be high, of course.) Hot and cold applications—another therapy I've seen used with great effect to moderate pain and to rid a body of toxicity. I saw a person receive this treatment for young adult schizophrenia (a condition that some authorities say can be a passing affliction). It took a few days with repeated applications on the back, but absolutely turned the corner. Do research this if you plan to try it, as the treatment was exacting and included other elements like doses of B vitamins, etc. Finally, don't forget foot baths, even if this is not the location of your pain, it can be done more easily and quickly than getting into a tub and has similar effects. Don't forget the Epsom salts!

Positional Therapies

Another strategy that helped my uncomfortable fibroid was putting my feet up the wall. I laid on my back with my rear end at the wall and legs extended upward. This did moderate pain for a while. Another positional therapy is the use of a raised head of the bed for GERD or reflux. After being miserable with the standard hard foam wedges advised for this condition, I discovered that several pillows arranged under my head, shoulders, and upper chest did the job without giving me neck and back aches that contended with the reflux symptoms for severity. Recommendations for digestive disorders also include lying on the left side—with promises that this is a pose less likely to cause reflux. Not sure about that, but it does feel a bit better. Conversely, when I've had heart "noise" (pain, palpitations, heaviness), I lie on my right side—which is recommended for heart issues.

Movement Therapies

After my life-threatening injury at 22 months old, I was put into a cast and then into a heavy brace with metal rods in it. I remember each being quite uncomfortable and frustratingly awkward. Doctors said I'd never use that leg again, drag it for the rest of my life, and experience nerve "ghost pains." The sole of my foot showed no nerve response to touch. My mother had taken Martha Graham dance classes and started me dancing daily to a record I still own with segments called Clown, Giant, Witch, Troll, and Fairy. I was to cavort as clown, stomp as giant and troll, swoop as witch, and flit as fairy. Actually, I stomped and flitted in a small circle with my dysfunctional leg in the center, being dragged and operating as a pivot point. As I got better, the circle got bigger. One year to the day of my injury, my mother's daily test of the bottom of my sole caused my toes to curl! The nerve had healed and the surgeon called it a medical miracle. Such things DO happen. I had a neighbor who was in a car accident where the seatbelt damaged her spine badly in a rollover accident. She was an adult but also recovered with the help of swimming. In 2006, one of my grand-daughters (then 18) was similarly injured and miraculously, several years later, began to have sensation again in a leg after a surgical procedure for a bed sore. Doctors have begun repairing her legs for eventual walking. Miracles DO happen. Movement can help. Hope definitely helps.

Self-Massage

My parents set the standard for my marriage—they gave/we give each other massages with some frequency. Those help with everything from sciatica to degenerating spinal discs, deteriorating joints, muscle spasms, insomnia, and migraines. After my father's death, in her senior years, my mother became a great proponent of self-massage. She was obese and had difficulty reaching to some spots, but she could do her own shoulders and head, and she could get to her feet. In the world of massage, feet are hugely significant as that is the main place where reflexology is done. The concept is that every spot on your body is represented by a spot on your feet. (Ears and hands have reflex points as well.) I became convinced that this was true when I discovered that the numb lowest part at the back of my big toe was the "thyroid" point, and I do have the familial problem with that important little endocrine gland. While any massage is better than none, I recommend downloading a chart and seeking out sore spots—seeing if they coordinate with problem body parts. Here is a link with a chart available to individuals for free http://www.pure-and-simple-healing.com/foot-reflexology-chart.html#.V63p4DUWwdU. Also, look up different kinds of strokes to do on a foot, but a finger doing circular motions feels great. Vary your pressure to discover what is best. Of course, if you have someone who will do massages or exchange them with you, that's a wonderful resource. Per sore knees, a naturopath told me that using a small (clean!) toilet bowl plunger brings helpful blood flow to the area. Always pay attention when massaging or being massaged—discomfort is NOT the goal.

Pain Medication

Most medications have side effects and can cause eventual harm if used for too long or in the wrong amounts. Use of pain medication is being called at epidemic proportions. My experience with migraines is that initially many things worked, then stopped working. Also, that some medications "call to themselves"—cause me to need more, sometimes by creating the symptom/s I was attempting to eliminate. Some things I've learned:

+ I would never suggest adamantly refusing medication as part of pain management. Even though I have so many alternative methods, I've used medication as well.

+ I use as little as I can and the gentlest form I can find, including herbs & homeopathics.

+ I rotate medicines when they lose potency. So, for example, the first dose for a headache, Ibuprofen. Second dose, acetaminophen. If a third dose is needed, aspirin.

 + I read pharmaceutical information packets so I'll know if I'm having a common reaction to a drug. I especially look for warnings about drugs that cause pain.

+ Rarely, do I use opiods like Vicodin as they literally cause me worsened pain after they wear off.

+ I seek to find and use other methods than drugs whenever possible. Drug use is not a "free ride" PERIOD. Example: Upping my magnesium intake has reduced my migraines.

Emotional Pain

Many of the strategies in this book work for emotional pains like sadness, depression, and fear as well as for physical pain. Sometimes, emotional pain causes physical pain and vice versa. Beyond those facts, I recommend *Mind Over Mood* for those with depression or anxiety. It's an easily understood and used workbook by Greenberger and Padesky.

Processing Loss Workbook is one I've written for people dealing with any kind of loss, including coping with pain, illness, or injury. It is available as an eBook http://www.amazon.com/dp/B017TZDBY0 or paperback http://www.amazon.com/dp/1519275080 through Amazon.

Talking about Pain

Of course, there are some times and places when we must clearly articulately describe our pain...to doctors, especially in emergency rooms, where over-estimating your pain level will get faster help than playing the brave stoic who gets left until everyone else has been helped. (Yes, I learned that by doing it.) Beyond that, caregivers whether family, friends, or hired help need some feedback about this symptom. As for the rest of the time, do yourself a favor and speak little to nothing about your pain. The less time you focus on pain, the better you'll be. The less people define you by your pain, the better your relationships will be. DO tell others how to relieve pain—methods you've found. I'm not suggesting, again, that you dummy up when you need help, simply that what you focus on expands, and how you define yourself influences how others and, most importantly, how you feel about yourself. Give yourself a break. Give others a break. Tell what you must on a need-to-know basis and find other topics to distract yourself. I've been known to teach through a migraine many times...often ending without it. I've taught a four-hour workshop after a car accident, and often sat down to the computer with some discomfort that left me while I worked and "got into the flow." If you want something to think and talk about, watch a funny movie, read an engaging book, find YouTubes of comic kittens/babies/puppies (slideshow of my kittens https://youtu.be/Z4-dRXmOPmI) , or indulge in making the world a better place. My book called *Gratitude* shares many of my favorite practices for making myself feel better like expressing gratitude or mentally telling everyone I see as I drive that I love them. Become an expert at planting flowers so that weeds don't have a place to grow. Best wishes & love to you. Let me know how these strategies work for you or about methods you've found: ariele@comcast.net.

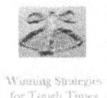

Making Mud Angels: Winning Strategies in ToughTimes http://www.amazon.com/dp/B00SOJD7M6 Need a fresh start? Help is here. Achieve success when finances, diet, health, or relationships are troubled. Easy Action Plans are gifts from tried and true wisdoms of the ages. Join the fun path to a better life. Paperback: http://www.amazon.com/dp/1507617070

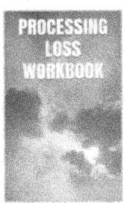

Processing Loss Workbook Whether it's a loved one, a pet, or your stock portfolio, loss can be depressing and painful. Worst of all, we often feel alone as we recover. In this unique workbook, you get to bring your loss with you: revel in previous good things, regret the change, feel accompanied in this journey, by those who understand— others who have experienced loss. (PS That's everybody!)
http://www.amazon.com/dp/B017TZDBY0
Paperback: http://www.amazon.com/dp/1519275080

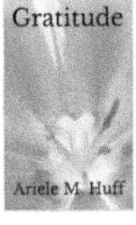

Gratitude http://www.amazon.com/dp/B01EWBMZZU A known restorative and tonic of mega proportions, being grateful is an art. Bring more into your life with these often humorous articles and short stories. It doesn't have to be Thanksgiving to enjoy giving thanks!

KITTEN LOVE: http://www.amazon.com/dp/B00OOHB068 Three kittens in

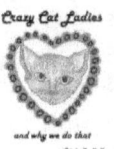

a box under a bush. What was I to do but take them home? In this game changing choice, I've learned a lot about myself, my husband, our two elderly pets, and how a single moment can make your life over --whether you wanted that or not! It's a raucous ride with melting moments and unbelievably adorable kittens. Plus, a couple of bumbling pet owners hoping to survive their best intentions. HELP!

Learn from My Mistakes http://www.amazon.com/dp/B00PLQNU0K An open diary of the happy, healing, humorous adventure—exploring obstacles and discovering solutions--bringing three abandoned kittens into our lives!

Crazy Cat Ladies and why we do that This is the story of how my husband and I graduated from lifetime owners of one-cat-at-a-time to Crazy Cat Ladies and why we love it so much. The answer is NOT what you think it is!

http://www.amazon.com/dp/B00V975HKG

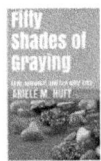

Fifty Shades of Graying: Love, Romance, and Sex After Fifty
http://www.amazon.com/dp/B00T85X2T4   The result of a blog
where people shared stories, essays, & poems on the topics.

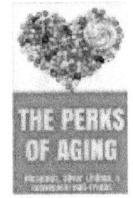

The Perks of Aging: Blessings, Silver Linings, & Convenient Half
Truths **eBook:** http://www.amazon.com/dp/B00VFAFAAE
Paper back: https://www.createspace.com/5399818

The Queen of Mean: The Conversion of a Cold and Prejudiced
Heart http://www.amazon.com/dp/B00TMCFPBG
A tattoo appears and comes to life, shocking a bitter bureaucrat
with letters in her own handwriting and nightly out-of-body
travel. True stories from immigrants and refugees mingle with
folktales and myths in a book that shows how spirits can bring magical
change—whether you want it or not! Fantasy novella.
Paperback: https://www.createspace.com/5408791

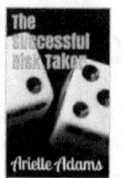

The Successful Risk Taker

http://www.amazon.com/dp/B00Y7PT366

What makes one person more prone to be a daredevil than another one? Why riding the risky but fun roller coaster, pushing limits, and love of adventure add up to the good life. A diary of childhood secrets and adult results. Roll the dice and win!

Kitten Love: The Trilogy The rescue of three fragile kittens, abandoned in a park. Their first months documented in three books, now forming a trilogy of touching, hectic, and illuminating journals of tiny lives...and the people and other pets affected by them. Challenges and lessons in love.

http://www.amazon.com/dp/B0167GEGFA

Paperback: https://www.createspace.com/5602517

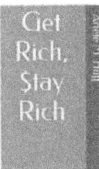

Get Rich, $tay Rich Make money your friend and servant. Learn the simple ways to becoming the richest person you know. This easy workbook is a step-by-step guide to bettering your life and your circumstances. Wealth is within your grasp.
http://www.amazon.com/dp/B012W5Z2W6 Also in paperback

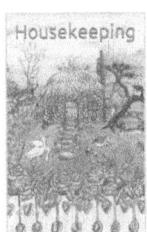

Housekeeping Anthology of essays about householding gathered since 1999. Funny and unexpectedly revealing.
http://www.amazon.com/dp/B01B3M4KW2 Also in paperback.

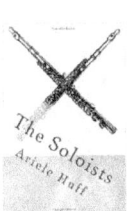

The Soloists Like child actors and athletes, musical child prodigies often pay a heavy price for their stardom. The people are real. All the situations and most of the events are real. This narrative nonfiction is written in novel form to document the lives of children placed into often brutal adult level competition, taking readers through the resulting emotional consequences. With a main character composited from two real life soloists, this novel is written by a family member.
https://www.amazon.com/dp/B01FNY5TO4

ABOUT THE AUTHOR

Ariele Huff hosts a website segment—Sharing Stories—on the LOCAL page of *Northwest Prime Time*. Contact: http://northwestprimetime.com

Columns Writing Corner and Poetry Corner are in the print version of *NW Prime Time* which is free at libraries and senior centers in Seattle and surrounding areas. Send your stories or poems for Sharing Stories or Poetry Corner to ariele@comcast.net.

Ariele teaches onsite writing classes in the Seattle area and online classes to people all over the world. Email for a complete list of class titles or with any writing questions.

Website for writers: http://arielewriter.myfreesites.net
Blog: http://writerswingsbyariele.blogspot.com/
Blog: http://fiftyshadesofgraying.blogspot.com/

BANDAID Books: a line of short, inexpensive, helpful eBooks and paperbacks meant to ease some particular difficulty, a friendly hand during an uncomfortable time.
Making Mud Angels: Winning Strategies in Tough Times
Processing Loss Workbook
PAIN: Treatments & Therapies

CANDY BAR Books: a line of short, sweet, and inexpensive eBooks and paperbacks meant to bring some pleasure—a laugh, a friendly face at the party, a snippet of wisdom.
Kitten Love: The Trilogy
Kitten Love
Learn from My Mistakes
Crazy Cat Ladies and Why We Do That
The Perks of Aging: Blessings, Silver Linings, & Convenient Half Truths
Gratitude
The Successful Risk Taker
The Queen of Mean: The Conversion of a Cold and Prejudiced Heart
Get Rich, $tay Rich
Fifty Shades of Graying: Love, Romance, and Sex After Fifty
The Last Duet
The Soloists

Ariele M. Huff

Ariele M. Huff